Carnivore Diet for Women

Grocery & Meal Planning Guide with 4 Tailored Plans for Weight Loss, Muscle Gain, Energy & Skin Health

copyright © 2025 Stephanie Hinderock

All rights reserved No part of this book may be reproduced, or stored in a retrieval system, or transmitted in any form or by any means, electronic, mechanical, photocopying, recording, or otherwise, without express written permission of the publisher.

Disclaimer

By reading this disclaimer, you are accepting the terms of the disclaimer in full. If you disagree with this disclaimer, please do not read the guide.

All of the content within this guide is provided for informational and educational purposes only, and should not be accepted as independent medical or other professional advice. The author is not a doctor, physician, nurse, mental health provider, or registered nutritionist/dietician. Therefore, using and reading this guide does not establish any form of a physician-patient relationship.

Always consult with a physician or another qualified health provider with any issues or questions you might have regarding any sort of medical condition. Do not ever disregard any qualified professional medical advice or delay seeking that advice because of anything you have read in this guide. The information in this guide is not intended to be any sort of medical advice and should not be used in lieu of any medical advice by a licensed and qualified medical professional.

The information in this guide has been compiled from a variety of known sources. However, the author cannot attest to or guarantee the accuracy of each source and thus should not be held liable for any errors or omissions.

You acknowledge that the publisher of this guide will not be held liable for any loss or damage of any kind incurred as a result of this guide or the reliance on any information provided within this guide. You acknowledge and agree that you assume all risk and responsibility for any action you undertake in response to the information in this guide.

Using this guide does not guarantee any particular result (e.g., weight loss or a cure). By reading this guide, you acknowledge that there are no guarantees to any specific outcome or results you can expect.

All product names, diet plans, or names used in this guide are for identification purposes only and are the property of their respective owners. The use of these names does not imply endorsement. All other trademarks cited herein are the property of their respective owners.

Where applicable, this guide is not intended to be a substitute for the original work of this diet plan and is, at most, a supplement to the original work for this diet plan and never a direct substitute. This guide is a personal expression of the facts of that diet plan.

Where applicable, persons shown in the cover images are stock photography models and the publisher has obtained the rights to use the images through license agreements with third-party stock image companies.

Table of Contents

Introduction	7
Understanding the Carnivore Diet	9
What Is the Carnivore Diet?	9
Principles of the Carnivore Diet	10
The Backbone of the Diet: Typical Foods Consumed	11
Why Meal Plans Are Essential for Success	13
Benefits of the Carnivore Diet for Women	14
Considerations and Potential Drawbacks	19
Carnivore Diet Grocery Shopping Guide	21
Best Sources for Quality Meats and Animal Products	21
Budget-Friendly Tips for Sourcing Grass-Fed Options	26
Prepping Your Pantry and Freezer for Success	32
Tools and Equipment	38
Must-Have Kitchen Tools for Carnivore Cooking	38
Meal Prep and Storage Tips	42
30-Day Carnivore Diet Weight Loss Meal Plan for Women	45
Portion Guidelines	45
Meal Plan Overview	46
Sample Recipes	49
Tips for Staying Motivated	53
30-Day High-Protein Carnivore Diet Muscle Building Meal Plan for Women	55
Nutrient Timing Strategies	55
Meal Plan Overview	56
Sample Recipes	61
Tips for Muscle Building Success	66
14-Day Carnivore Diet Meal Plan for Energy and Focus	68
Key Nutrients for Energy and Focus	68
Meal Guidelines for Busy Professionals	69

14-Day Meal Plan	70
Quick Recipes for Busy Days	75
Final Tips for Energy and Focus	80

21-Day Carnivore Diet Meal Plan for Anti-Aging and Skin Health — 81

Key Nutrients for Anti-Aging and Glowing Skin	81
Tips for Reducing Sugar-Induced Skin Aging	82
21-Day Anti-Aging Meal Plan	83
Recipes for Skin Health	89
Final Tips for Glowing Skin	92

Inspiring Success Stories from Women on the Carnivore Diet — 93

Judy	93
Alisha Khan	93
Barb Shaw	94

Conclusion — 95
FAQs — 98
References and Helpful Links — 101

Introduction

When it comes to organizing a meal plan, simplicity often becomes elusive in the shuffle of endless options. For women looking to redefine their approach to food by cutting out the extras and focusing on a streamlined diet, this Carnivore Meal Plan and Grocery Guide offers a clear path forward. By narrowing decisions down to a selection of nutrient-packed essentials, it aims to change how meals are prepared, enjoyed, and sourced.

In this guide, we will talk about the following:

- Understanding The Carnivore Diet
- Carnivore Diet Grocery Shopping Guide
- Must-Have Kitchen Tools and Equipment for Women on the Carnivore Diet
- 30-Day Carnivore Diet Weight Loss Meal Plan for Women
- 30-Day High-Protein Carnivore Diet Muscle Building Meal Plan for Women
- 14-Day Carnivore Diet Meal Plan for Energy and Focus

- 21-Day Carnivore Diet Meal Plan for Anti-Aging and Skin Health

The meal plan itself breaks things down into manageable steps, covering what works for breakfast, lunch, dinner, and even snacks. Whether meals are cooked in batches for convenience or prepared fresh each time, this approach adapts to different lifestyles. All the guesswork has been removed, making it easy to stay consistent.

Keep reading to learn more about crafting meals that fit this straightforward style and stocking a kitchen with only the essentials. By the end of this guide, you'll have everything needed to feel empowered in the kitchen and on the path to optimal health and wellness.

Understanding the Carnivore Diet

The Carnivore Diet represents a bold and highly unconventional approach to eating. Its principle is as straightforward as it is radical—consume only animal-based foods while eliminating all forms of plant-derived products.

This simplicity appeals to those who want a clear-cut nutritional framework while also tapping into a way of eating that some believe mirrors the diet of our ancestors. However, with its restrictive nature and lack of variety, the Carnivore Diet requires careful consideration, planning, and a clear understanding of its benefits and challenges.

What Is the Carnivore Diet?

At its core, the Carnivore Diet is a zero-carbohydrate dietary plan that focuses exclusively on animal-based foods. This includes meat, fish, eggs, and animal fats, sometimes complemented by dairy products for those who do not experience sensitivity to lactose or casein.

No plant-based foods are allowed—this means no grains, fruits, vegetables, legumes, nuts, or seeds. Even oils derived from plants, such as olive and avocado oil, are off-limits.

The Carnivore Diet can be seen as an extreme evolution of ketogenic and low-carb diets. By eliminating carbohydrates entirely, it encourages the body to rely on fat, rather than glucose, as its primary energy source. This metabolic state, known as ketosis, is believed to provide more stable energy levels and reduce blood sugar fluctuations.

Principles of the Carnivore Diet

The principles of the carnivore diet, particularly for women, focus on consuming animal-based foods while eliminating plant-based foods. Here are the core principles:

1. ***Animal-Based Foods:*** The diet primarily consists of meat, fish, eggs, and animal-derived products like bone marrow and animal fats. Some variations include dairy, but this depends on individual tolerance.
2. ***Elimination of Plant Foods:*** All plant-based foods, including fruits, vegetables, grains, nuts, and seeds, are excluded. The focus is on reducing carbohydrates and fiber intake.
3. ***Focus on Nutrient Density:*** Emphasis is placed on consuming nutrient-dense animal products to meet nutritional needs, including essential vitamins and minerals.

4. ***Simplicity and Satiety:*** Meals are simple, often consisting of a single type of meat or a combination of animal products. The diet aims to promote satiety and reduce cravings.
5. ***Listening to the Body:*** Women are encouraged to listen to their bodies and eat when hungry, focusing on natural hunger cues rather than following a strict eating schedule.
6. ***Hydration and Electrolytes:*** Adequate hydration and maintaining electrolyte balance are important, as the diet can lead to changes in water retention and mineral balance.
7. ***Individual Adaptation:*** The diet may be adjusted based on individual health goals, activity levels, and personal preferences, allowing for some flexibility within the animal-based framework.

These principles guide the carnivore diet's approach, aiming to simplify food choices and focus on animal-derived nutrition.

The Backbone of the Diet: Typical Foods Consumed

The Carnivore Diet is strictly centered on foods derived from animals. These are more than just the staples of every meal—they are the only foods consumed on this dietary regimen. Here's a closer look at what's typically included:

- *Meat:* Various cuts of beef, pork, lamb, chicken, and turkey form the foundation. Organ meats like liver, heart, and kidney are often highlighted for their high vitamin and mineral content, including iron, B vitamins, and vitamin A.
- *Seafood:* Fish such as salmon, mackerel, and sardines, along with shellfish like shrimp, crab, and oysters, provide rich sources of omega-3 fatty acids and other nutrients.
- *Eggs:* Both whole eggs and egg yolks are highly valued for their healthy fats, protein, and micronutrient density.
- *Animal Fats:* Tallow (beef fat), lard (pork fat), butter, and ghee (clarified butter) provide essential calories and make meals more satisfying.
- *Optional Dairy (if tolerated):* Some individuals include cheese, cream, and yogurt made from milk. However, full-fat, low-carbohydrate options are encouraged to maintain the zero-carb goal.

Among devotees, grass-fed, pasture-raised meats and wild-caught seafood are often preferred for their quality and nutrient profiles. Ethical considerations and environmental impact further influence these choices.

Why Meal Plans Are Essential for Success

Transitioning to the Carnivore Diet isn't just about eating meat—it requires careful planning. Developing a meal plan is crucial to ensure you're meeting your nutritional needs and sticking to the diet without falling back into old habits.

Meal plans help:

1. **Prevent Nutritional Gaps**

   While sticking to an animal-based diet, it's crucial to include a variety of nutrient-rich foods to avoid deficiencies. For example, fatty fish like salmon or mackerel provide essential omega-3 fatty acids, which are vital for brain function and heart health.

   Similarly, organ meats such as liver are packed with vitamins like A and B12, which support energy production, immune health, and vision. Diversifying your protein sources ensures your body gets the full range of nutrients it needs to thrive.

2. **Avoid Monotony**

   Eating steak for every meal might sound appealing at first, especially if you're a meat lover, but the repetition can quickly lead to boredom. This monotony can make it harder to stick with the diet over time.

   Meal plans that incorporate different cuts of meat, such as lamb chops, pork belly, or chicken thighs, can add variety. Exploring different cooking methods like grilling, slow roasting, or sous-vide can also keep meals interesting and enjoyable, helping you stay motivated and excited about your diet.

3. **Stay on Track**

   Following an animal-based diet without a clear plan can make things more challenging. Without structure, you may face decision fatigue, where choosing what to eat feels overwhelming, or you might unintentionally derail your progress with unbalanced meals.

   A well-thought-out meal plan simplifies your daily routine, ensuring you prepare meals ahead of time and effectively balance your protein and fat intake. By staying organized, you can maintain consistency and achieve your dietary goals more easily.

By taking the time to map out your weekly meals, you'll set yourself up for long-term success on the Carnivore Diet.

Benefits of the Carnivore Diet for Women

While the Carnivore Diet can benefit anyone, women may experience unique advantages. Here's how:

1. **Potential Hormonal Balance**

   Hormonal health is essential for women's well-being, but imbalances can cause issues like irregular cycles,

PCOS, or mood swings. The Carnivore Diet may support hormone production and regulation through its focus on animal-based fats and proteins.

- *Animal Fats for Hormone Production:* Hormones like estrogen, progesterone, and testosterone are made from cholesterol, found in foods like butter, egg yolks, and fatty meats. Eating these fats provides the body with the building blocks for balanced hormones.
- *Reduced Insulin Spikes:* Processed carbs and sugars cause blood sugar swings and insulin spikes, which can disrupt hormones and worsen PCOS. Cutting these foods helps stabilize blood sugar and supports hormonal balance.
- *Improved Menstrual Regularity:* Many women on this diet report more regular cycles and less PMS. This may be due to balanced blood sugar and reduced inflammation, both important for hormonal health.

This focus on hormonal balance isn't just physical—it extends to emotional well-being, offering mood stability and helping combat the anxiety and irritability tied to imbalanced hormones. For women seeking a natural approach to hormonal health, the Carnivore Diet provides a promising avenue.

2. Improved Weight Management

One of the most immediate and noticeable benefits of the Carnivore Diet for women is its impact on weight management. Whether the goal is to lose weight or maintain a healthy one, this diet offers several advantages that make it easier to achieve these goals.

- ***Satiety and Reduced Hunger:*** Animal-based foods are nutrient-dense, providing more vitamins and minerals with fewer calories. Foods like steak, eggs, and fatty fish are filling, helping prevent overeating or snacking.
- ***Fewer Cravings:*** Cutting out sugary foods and carbs reduces blood sugar spikes, stabilizing appetite and curbing junk food cravings.
- ***Fat Adaptation and Energy Use:*** The Carnivore Diet trains the body to use fat for energy instead of carbs, improving fat-burning and supporting steady weight loss or maintenance without extreme calorie cutting.

For women who feel like they've "tried everything," the simplicity of meat and animal-based foods removes the mental and physical hurdles that come with calorie counting and constant hunger. Weight loss feels less like deprivation and more like building a sustainable relationship with food.

3. **Energy and Mental Clarity**

   Modern diets filled with processed carbs and sugary snacks often leave people cycling between energy highs and debilitating slumps. On the Carnivore Diet, many women report consistent energy levels throughout the day and a dramatic increase in mental clarity.

   - *Consistent Energy:* Without the roller-coaster of blood sugar spikes and crashes, the body can maintain steady energy throughout the day. Fat and protein provide slow-burning fuel, keeping you energized for hours after a meal.
   - *Reduction in Brain Fog:* Many women transitioning to the Carnivore Diet notice an improvement in mental clarity and focus. Removing inflammatory plant compounds and sugars can reduce cognitive sluggishness, leaving the brain better-equipped to handle stress and workload.
   - *Promoting Better Sleep:* Improved hormonal balance and the absence of energy-disrupting foods can also lead to better-quality sleep, which further contributes to how alert and sharp you feel during the day.

   For busy women juggling careers, families, or other commitments, this boost in consistent energy and mental sharpness can make a tangible difference in daily life.

4. **Improved Skin and Joint Health**

   Chronic inflammation plays a significant role in many women's health concerns, including acne flare-ups and stubborn joint pain. By eliminating plant-based components like oxalates and lectins, the Carnivore Diet may help reduce these issues.

   - *Clearer Skin:* Acne is often linked to inflammation and hormonal imbalances. By stabilizing hormones and cutting out inflammatory foods, many women experience healthier, clearer complexions. Additionally, the collagen found in animal products like bone broth or gelatin supports skin elasticity and hydration.
   - *Reduced Joint Pain:* Vegetables like spinach, kale, and peppers might seem healthy but can contain oxalates—compounds that could contribute to joint inflammation in sensitive individuals. On a Carnivore Diet, the absence of oxalates may ease symptoms of arthritis or other joint discomfort.
   - *Anti-Inflammatory Effects of Animal-Based Foods:* Omega-3-rich foods like salmon also

play a crucial role in reducing inflammation, further benefiting both skin and joint health.

The Carnivore Diet's focus on unprocessed, nutrient-dense animal products can provide numerous health benefits for women. However, as with any dietary change, it's essential to consult a healthcare professional before making significant adjustments to your eating habits.

Considerations and Potential Drawbacks

While proponents emphasize the Carnivore Diet's simplicity and benefits, acknowledging its challenges is crucial for providing a balanced perspective:

- *Restrictive Nature:* Cutting out all plant-based foods can feel monotonous or socially isolating. Dining out or attending gatherings may pose difficulties due to the lack of compliant options.
- *Risk of Nutrient Deficiencies:* Without meal planning, there's the potential to miss out on nutrients such as vitamin C, fiber, or magnesium, which are abundant in plant-based foods.
- *Adaptation Phase:* Many individuals experience a transitional period of fatigue, digestive changes, and cravings as the body adjusts to running on fats instead of carbs.

- ***Ethical and Environmental Questions:*** The heavy reliance on animal products may raise concerns for those mindful of ethical or sustainability issues.

Despite these factors, the Carnivore Diet continues to gain popularity among women seeking an alternative approach to nutrition. However, it's essential to consult with a healthcare professional before embarking on any dietary changes and assess whether this diet aligns with your individual health goals and needs.

Carnivore Diet Grocery Shopping Guide

Transitioning to the Carnivore Diet is more than just a shift in what you eat—it's a full transformation of how you shop, stock, and prepare your food. With the focus entirely on animal-based products, grocery shopping requires strategic planning to ensure your meals are both high-quality and aligned with your budget. This chapter will help you shop smarter, keep costs down, and organize your kitchen to support long-term success on the Carnivore Diet.

Best Sources for Quality Meats and Animal Products

The foundation of the Carnivore Diet is high-quality animal products. Prioritizing nutrient-rich foods from well-raised animals can make a significant difference in both health benefits and flavor. Here's how to get the best products:

1. **Local Butchers**

    Local butchers are often your best bet for sourcing fresh, high-quality meat. Many butcher shops work directly with nearby farms, allowing you to access pasture-raised and grass-fed options. The benefits include:

- ***Customization:*** Butchers offer personalized service, allowing you to request specific cuts, organ meats, or bones for broths—customization that's hard to find in supermarkets.
- ***Freshness:*** Butchers provide fresher, higher-quality meat by sourcing directly from local farms and suppliers, often just days after processing, unlike pre-packaged options stored for weeks.
- ***Advice:*** Butchers are meat experts who offer cooking tips and guidance on using various cuts, helping you elevate your meals.

2. **Farmers' Markets**

Farmers' markets provide a direct link to the source. Shopping here allows you to educate yourself about farming practices while supporting local farmers. Key advantages include:

- ***Transparency:*** Farmers' markets give you the chance to speak directly with the farmers about how they raise their animals or grow their produce. This personal connection helps ensure that your food is sourced ethically and sustainably, giving you peace of mind about what you're buying.

- ***Unique Products:*** Unlike supermarkets, farmers' markets often feature specialty items you won't find elsewhere. From pasture-raised eggs and wild-caught fish to freshly rendered lard and hand-crafted cheeses, these markets are a treasure trove of unique, high-quality products that stand out for their freshness and flavor.

- ***Seasonal Deals:*** Shopping at the right time can also save you money. Many farmers offer discounts toward the end of the market day to sell off their remaining stock, or during certain seasons when specific produce is in abundance. It's a great opportunity to stock up on fresh, local goods while supporting small-scale farmers.

3. Online Meat Providers

If you live in an area with limited access to specialty stores or farmers' markets, online retailers are a convenient option. Many companies specialize in delivering grass-fed, organic, and pasture-raised products nationwide. Consider these tips:

- ***Reputation Matters:*** Look for companies with strong customer reviews and a proven track record of transparency about where and how their meat is sourced. Ethical practices and high-quality sourcing can make a big difference in the taste and health benefits of the meat.

- *Bundle Deals:* Many online providers offer cost-effective bulk packages, such as "family boxes" or mixed meat subscriptions, which allow you to save money while trying a variety of cuts and types of meat. These bundles are perfect for families or anyone looking to meal prep.
- *Frozen Benefits:* Meats are typically delivered frozen, which locks in nutrients and flavor while ensuring long-term freshness. This makes it easy to store and use over time without worrying about spoilage, especially if your schedule varies.

4. **Grocery Stores**

While supermarket chains may lack personalized options, they can still be a reliable source for Carnivore staples. Seek out:

- *Grass-Fed & Organic Sections:* Many grocery stores now offer organic and grass-fed meats in their specialty aisles, providing a healthier and more sustainable choice for consumers. These options are typically free from added hormones

or antibiotics, making them a favorite for those prioritizing clean eating.
- *Wild-Caught Fish:* High-quality seafood options like salmon, mackerel, or cod are often found in the frozen section. Wild-caught fish is prized for its natural flavor and higher nutritional value compared to farmed alternatives, offering a great source of omega-3 fatty acids.
- *Pasture-Raised Eggs & Butter:* Look for these in the organic dairy aisle, where you can find items labeled "pasture-raised" or "grass-fed." Pasture-raised eggs come from hens that roam freely, producing eggs with richer yolks, while grass-fed butter is known for its creamy texture and higher levels of beneficial fats.

Decoding Labels for Quality

Not all labels are created equal. Here's what to look for to ensure you're getting the best quality:

- *Grass-Fed vs. Grass-Finished:* "Grass-fed" means the animal started its diet on grass but may have been finished on grains to fatten them up before processing. In contrast, "grass-finished" ensures the animal ate grass its entire life, resulting in leaner meat with a distinct flavor profile.

- ***Pasture-Raised:*** Indicates animals were raised with access to pasture, allowing them to roam freely and graze naturally, unlike animals typically confined to small spaces in industrial farming. This often results in higher-quality meat and eggs with better nutritional value.
- ***Certified Organic:*** Guarantees the animal was raised without synthetic hormones, antibiotics, or genetically modified feed. It also ensures humane living conditions and is regulated under strict USDA standards.
- ***Wild-caught (for seafood):*** This means the fish were caught in their natural environment, such as oceans, rivers, or lakes, rather than raised in crowded fish farms. Wild-caught seafood often has a more natural diet and is considered more sustainable when sourced responsibly.

Budget-Friendly Tips for Sourcing Grass-Fed Options

Grass-fed meat is often considered the gold standard for the Carnivore Diet, offering superior taste, nutritional benefits, and ethical sourcing. However, it can be pricey, making it tough to fit into everyday budgets. Luckily, with smart strategies and a little planning, you can enjoy high-quality, grass-fed options without breaking the bank. Here's how:

1. **Buy in Bulk**

   Purchasing meat in bulk is one of the most cost-effective ways to include grass-fed options in your diet.

   - ***Local Farms:*** Many farms sell whole or half portions of animals like beef or lamb directly to consumers. Not only is this cheaper per pound than buying individual cuts, but it also guarantees traceable and sustainable sourcing.
   - ***CSA Programs:*** Community-Supported Agriculture (CSA) programs often allow you to purchase a share of a farm's production, which can include grass-fed meat. Look for programs in your area that offer customizable boxes to match your preferences.
   - ***Shared Purchases:*** If buying a half or full cow seems overwhelming, consider splitting the purchase with friends or family. This keeps costs down while still reaping the savings of bulk buying.

2. **Visit Local Farmers' Markets**

   Farmers' markets are treasure troves for discovering affordable grass-fed and pasture-raised meats.

   - ***Ask About Deals:*** Farmers often sell cuts that are less known (and less expensive), such as oxtail, brisket, or organ meats, which are still nutritious and versatile.

- **Build Relationships:** Get to know your local farmers; they may offer discounts for repeat customers or notify you of upcoming sales.
- **End-of-Day Discounts:** Visit the market toward closing time to score deals on products that the vendors don't want to pack and haul back.

3. **Explore Online Options**

The internet offers a range of options for sourcing grass-fed meats at competitive prices.

- **Specialty Meat Suppliers:** Websites like ButcherBox, US Wellness Meats, and others deliver high-quality grass-fed meats straight to your door. Many of these services offer affordable subscription boxes with bulk savings.
- **Online Farms:** Some farms have their own websites where you can purchase directly. These sites often include details about how the animals are raised, giving you transparency along with savings.
- **Flash Sales and Coupons:** Watch for special promotions, free shipping offers, or discounts for first-time buyers when shopping online.

4. **Prioritize Quality on a Budget**

   Stretching your dollar without sacrificing quality means understanding where to compromise and where to focus your spending.

   - *Choose Ground Meat:* Ground beef is often one of the cheapest ways to enjoy grass-fed options. It's versatile and works for almost any meal, from burgers to casseroles.
   - *Go for Lesser-Known Cuts:* Opt for cuts like shank, chuck roast, or brisket. These are often cheaper than steaks but just as nutritious. When cooked properly (e.g., slow cooking or braising), they're tender and full of flavor.
   - *Mix and Match:* If 100% grass-fed isn't feasible, consider mixing it with conventionally raised meat. For example, use grass-fed ground beef in your main dishes while supplementing with regular options for sides or snacks.

5. **Plan Meals and Use Leftovers Efficiently**

   Planning ahead is key to getting the most out of your grass-fed purchases. Every dollar counts, so minimizing waste is essential.

   - *Batch Cooking:* Cook large portions of meat at once and portion them into meals for the week. This not only saves time but also ensures you're using your grass-fed meat wisely.

- ***Bone Broth:*** Save bones from roasts or steaks to make nutrient-rich bone broth. This extends the value of your meat and creates a flavorful base for soups or beverages.
- ***Freeze Extras:*** Properly store and freeze grass-fed meats to maintain freshness. Invest in a vacuum sealer or freezer bags to prevent freezer burn and extend the shelf life of larger purchases.

6. **Get Creative with Meal Prep**

Making the most of affordable cuts often means getting a little creative in the kitchen.

- ***Slow Cookers and Braising:*** Tougher, cheaper cuts like brisket or short ribs become meltingly tender when slow-cooked. These methods also allow you to cook in bulk.
- ***Carnivore Staples from Scraps:*** Turn leftover meat trimmings into snack-friendly items like carnivore jerky or crispy cracklings.
- ***Add Variety:*** Mix up your meal prep with different animal sources. Grass-fed pork or lamb, for example, is often more budget-friendly than beef.

7. **Be Strategic About Storage**

   Proper storage ensures that nothing goes to waste, especially when you're investing in high-quality grass-fed meats.

   - *Use a Deep Freezer:* If you're buying in bulk, investing in a deep freezer is a must. It lets you freeze large quantities without running out of space in your regular freezer.
   - *Label and Rotate:* Keep track of what's in your freezer by labeling packages with dates. Rotate older cuts to the front to use first and prevent spoilage.
   - *Portion Wisely:* When freezing bulk purchases, divide meats into meal-sized portions. This makes defrosting faster and helps you take out only what you need.

Why Grass-Fed Matters

Grass-fed meat isn't just a trendy choice—it offers tangible benefits worth prioritizing.

- *Nutritional Superiority:* Grass-fed beef boasts greater amounts of Omega-3 fatty acids, conjugated linoleic acid (CLA), and essential vitamins such as A and E when compared to its grain-fed counterpart.
- *Ethical and Sustainable Farming Practices:* Grass-fed farms often follow eco-friendly and

animal-friendly practices, which support sustainable agriculture.

While sourcing grass-fed meat can seem costly upfront, these budget-friendly strategies make it possible to enjoy the benefits without overspending. With careful planning, smart shopping, and creative cooking, you can maintain both your commitment to the Carnivore Diet and your household budget.

Prepping Your Pantry and Freezer for Success

Getting organized is crucial when starting the Carnivore Diet. Ensuring your pantry, freezer, and kitchen are well-stocked and streamlined will make it easier to stay consistent and eliminate mealtime stress. Below, we'll cover how to prep and organize your pantry and freezer effectively, the must-have items to include, proper storage techniques, and meal planning tips to set you up for success.

Stocking Your Pantry with Carnivore Essentials

While the Carnivore Diet focuses on fresh and frozen animal-based foods, your pantry can still play a supporting role. Here are some essential items to keep on hand:

1. **Animal Fats and Cooking Oils**
    - Tallow, lard, duck fat, and butter are staples for cooking and flavor. These shelf-stable fats

provide a quick energy source and are ideal for searing and frying.
- Keep these fats in airtight containers, stored in a cool, dark place to maintain freshness.

2. **Bone Broth and Gelatin**
   - Stock up on high-quality, ready-made bone broths or make your own and store it in jars. This is perfect for sipping or as a base for carnivore-friendly meals.
   - Gelatin powder made from animal sources can also be a great addition to support joint and skin health.

3. **Salt and Seasonings**
   - Invest in high-quality salts like Himalayan pink salt or Redmond salt. These provide essential minerals that help balance electrolytes.
   - Avoid packaged seasoning blends with added sugar—stick to simple, carnivore-friendly spices like black pepper or dried herbs if tolerated.

4. **Shelf-Stable Extras**
   - Canned fish (e.g., sardines, mackerel, tuna) in water or olive oil serve as quick and portable protein options.
   - Dehydrated meats or carnivore-friendly jerky with no additives are great for snacking and travel.

Freezer Prep for Carnivore Diet Success

Your freezer will quickly become the backbone of your kitchen on the Carnivore Diet. Here's how to prepare and organize it for easy access and optimal freshness:

1. **Stock a Variety of Meats**
   - Include a mix of beef, pork, poultry, lamb, and seafood. Ground meat is a versatile, budget-friendly option, while steaks and roasts offer variety. Don't forget nutrient-dense organ meats like liver or kidney.
   - Store individual portions to avoid defrosting more than you need for a single meal. Vacuum sealing or freezer-safe bags work best for preventing freezer burn.

2. **Freeze Pre-Cooked Meals**
   - Batch cook dishes like shredded beef, braised short ribs, or carnivore burgers, and freeze them in individual containers for quick meals.
   - Label containers with the contents and date to ensure nothing gets lost at the back of the freezer.

3. **Portion Animal Fats:** Freeze butter or rendered animal fats in ice cube trays for convenient single-use servings. This prevents waste and keeps your diet streamlined.

4. **Bone Storage:** Save bones from roasts or steaks for making broth. Store them in a dedicated freezer bag labeled for this purpose.

Creating a Carnivore-Friendly Kitchen Environment

A well-organized kitchen is essential for sticking to your dietary goals. Make your kitchen a space that supports your carnivore lifestyle with these tips:

1. **Organize by Zones**
   - Dedicate sections in your refrigerator, freezer, and pantry exclusively to carnivore foods. This keeps your ingredients separate and easy to find.
   - Use clear bins or labeled containers to store similar items together—for example, one bin in the fridge for cooked meats and another for fresh cuts or deli items.
2. **Invest in Essential Tools**
   - A slow cooker, instant pot, or air fryer will simplify cooking tougher cuts of meat like brisket or short ribs.
   - Sharp knives and a quality cutting board are crucial for prepping meats efficiently. Consider a meat thermometer to cook large cuts precisely.
   - Vacuum sealers are ideal for storing bulk meat purchases and preventing spoilage.

3. **Declutter and Purge Unfriendly Items:** Remove temptation by clearing out non-carnivore foods. Donate pantry staples like grains or legumes to reduce clutter and make space for animal-based essentials.

Meal Planning and Batch Cooking Tips

Planning ahead is key to making the Carnivore Diet manageable, especially if you're busy. Batch cooking and meal prep will save you time, reduce food waste, and ensure you always have compliant meals ready to go.

1. **Plan Weekly Menus:** Decide on staple meals for the week—like steak and eggs or slow-cooked roasts. Having a clear plan helps you buy only what you need and avoid mid-week grocery runs.
2. **Batch Cook Basics**
   - Prepare large quantities of commonly used foods like ground beef, roasted chicken, or bacon. Portion them into containers and refrigerate or freeze for easy reheating.
   - Cook extras for easy leftovers. For example, make a double batch of broth or braised meats to span several meals.
3. **Use Every Part of Your Ingredients:**
   - Save meat drippings, like bacon grease, for cooking other dishes.
   - Turn leftover meat scraps into snacks like carnivore crisps or jerky to avoid waste.

4. **<u>Set Aside Time for Prep</u>:** Dedicate one or two days a week to prepping and cooking. For example, Sunday can be your batch cooking day to fill your fridge and freezer with ready-to-eat meals for the week.

Prepping your pantry and freezer is about more than just organization—it's about creating a supportive, hassle-free kitchen environment that makes it easy to stick to your Carnivore Diet goals. When your essentials are stocked, your meals are planned, and your kitchen is efficient, you'll set yourself up for long-term success while keeping stress at a minimum.

Tools and Equipment

Being well-equipped in the kitchen can transform your carnivore cooking experience from overwhelming to effortless. Whether you're searing the perfect steak, slow-cooking tender ribs, or prepping a week's worth of meals, the right tools and techniques can help you nail the flavor and texture every time. In this chapter, we'll cover essential kitchen tools for any meat-lover's arsenal and share some practical tips for prepping and storing your carnivorous feasts.

Must-Have Kitchen Tools for Carnivore Cooking

In addition to basic kitchen staples like a chef's knife and cutting board, here are some essential tools that will make your carnivore cooking experience more efficient and enjoyable:

1. **Cast Iron Skillet**

    A cast iron skillet is a must. It's versatile, durable, and perfect for achieving that golden-brown crust on meats. Cast iron conducts heat evenly, making it ideal for searing, frying, and even baking dishes like meat pies or carnivore-friendly quiches. Plus, with proper care and seasoning, these skillets become nearly nonstick and last a lifetime.

Tip: Make sure your skillet is preheated for a few minutes before adding the meat. This helps lock in juices and flavor.

2. **Sharp Knives**

   A sharp knife isn't just a luxury—it's a necessity. Dull blades can tear meat fibers and make slicing harder, resulting in uneven cuts and less professional plating. Invest in a good chef's knife for general prep and a boning knife for trimming fat and cleaning bones.

   Pro Tip: Regularly hone your knives to maintain their edge and consider sharpening them professionally a few times a year if you're cooking a lot of meat.

3. **Meat Thermometer**

   To achieve perfectly cooked meat, a reliable meat thermometer is non-negotiable. Internal temperatures matter whether you're grilling steak, roasting chicken, or smoking brisket. Guessing when meat is done can lead to dry or undercooked results, but with a thermometer, you'll always hit your target.

Quick Guide to Temps:

- Medium-rare steak: 130-135°F
- Chicken breast (fully cooked): 165°F
- Pork loin (juicy and safe): 145°F

4. Heavy-Duty Tongs

Tongs are a workhorse tool for any meat-focused cook. They allow you to flip steaks, move roasts, and toss cooked meat without puncturing it, which helps retain juices. Look for a sturdy, stainless steel set with a good grip.

5. Cutting Boards

A large cutting board dedicated to raw meat is essential. Plastic boards are great for easy cleaning and less risk of cross-contamination. Alternatively, heavy wooden butcher blocks work well for carving cooked cuts. Having separate boards for raw meat and cooked food is highly recommended for maintaining food safety.

6. Vacuum Sealer

If you're serious about meal prep or buying bulk, a vacuum sealer is a game-changer. Sealing meat removes excess air, extending its freezer life and preserving quality. It's also invaluable for sous vide cooking, ensuring your meat cooks evenly in its sealed bag.

7. **Sheet Trays and Wire Racks**

   Sheet trays are perfect for roasting or broiling meat, while wire racks add extra versatility by allowing heat to circulate around your meat for even cooking. They're also handy for resting meat or draining grease.

8. **Slow Cooker or Instant Pot**

   For tender, fall-apart cuts of meat like pork shoulder, short ribs, or brisket, a slow cooker or Instant Pot is a lifesaver. These appliances simplify the process and can save you hours of active cooking time.

9. **Kitchen Shears**

   Sturdy kitchen shears can handle jobs that knives struggle with, such as trimming fat, spatchcocking a chicken, or slicing through tough packaging. Some shears even come apart, making cleanup easy.

10. **Grill or Broiler Pan**

    Carnivore cooking often calls for the smoky char and sizzle that only a grill can deliver. If you don't have an outdoor grill, a broiler pan can mimic similar results indoors. Look for one that's durable and easy to clean.

With the right tools, cooking meat can be both enjoyable and efficient. These essential items will not only make your life easier in the kitchen but also help you get the most out of your meat.

Meal Prep and Storage Tips

Now that you have the tools to cook delicious meat, here are some tips for meal prep and storage to keep your meals safe and flavorful:

1. **Portioning for Success**

    When working with large cuts of meat, portion them right after purchase. Divide whole roasts, ribs, or packs of steaks into smaller servings before freezing. This makes it much easier to thaw only what you need instead of defrosting an entire pack. For a one-person household, individual portions work best. For families, package batch-friendly amounts.

    Tip: Write the portion size and date on your storage bags so you can keep track of what's in your freezer.

2. **Freezing Meat Properly**

    Freezer burn is a carnivore's enemy. To avoid it, use airtight packaging. Vacuum sealers work best, but good-quality freezer bags can also do the job. If using bags, press out as much air as possible before sealing them. You can also double-wrap cuts in plastic wrap and foil for added protection.

    For the best texture and flavor, use frozen meat within 3-6 months, depending on the type. Lean cuts like chicken breast may last longer, while fatty cuts like pork belly are best used sooner.

3. **Quick Thawing Tips**

   The safest way to thaw meat is to transfer it from the freezer to the fridge overnight. If you're in a hurry, submerge the sealed bag in a bowl of cold water, changing the water every 30 minutes. Avoid using hot water or leaving meat on the countertop, as this can promote bacterial growth.

4. **Batch Cooking for Efficiency**

   Prepping large batches of cooked meat can be a lifesaver during busy weeks. Cook a dozen burgers, roast a big pork shoulder, or grill several steaks at once. Store them in the fridge in individual portions so they're ready to reheat.

   Ideas: Sliced steak makes great toppings for fried eggs, shredded beef works perfectly in lettuce wraps, and crispy bacon is always a good snack or garnish.

5. **Storing Leftovers**

   Once cooked, store leftovers in small, airtight containers to keep them fresh and juicy. Avoid letting meat sit in its own juices; use paper towels or separate the meat with wax paper for better texture. Refrigerated cooked meat typically lasts 3-4 days, while properly stored frozen leftovers can last up to 2-3 months.

6. **Marinades and Spice Blends**

   If you're marinating, consider preparing spice blends and marinades in bulk and storing them in jars. Meat can even be frozen directly in its marinade, so when it thaws, it's already flavorful and ready to cook.

Having the right tools and storage strategies can revolutionize how you approach the carnivore diet. With a well-stocked kitchen and some thoughtful prep, you'll save time, reduce waste, and always have delicious, high-quality meals at your fingertips.

30-Day Carnivore Diet Weight Loss Meal Plan for Women

This 30-day carnivore meal plan is designed to help women lose fat, stay energized, and feel satisfied. It focuses on high-quality animal-based products, portion control, and a structured approach to ensure steady progress. The daily meals are lightweight but nutrient-dense, ensuring you don't compromise on essential nutrients.

Portion Guidelines

Calorie needs vary based on activity level, age, and weight. A general guideline for fat loss on the carnivore diet is to consume **1 gram of protein per pound of ideal body weight** and include high-quality fats for energy. Use these portions as a starting point and adjust based on hunger, energy, and results.

- *Protein:* 4–6 oz per meal (about the size of your palm)
- *Fat:* Add a thumb-sized portion of butter, tallow, or lard, if needed

- *Calories:* Aim for a slight caloric deficit (subtract ~300–500 calories from your maintenance level)

Meal Plan Overview

Below is a daily structure to simplify meal planning. Each day includes Breakfast, Lunch, Dinner, and optional Snacks if you need more energy.

- *Breakfast:* Simple, protein-rich start
- *Lunch:* Moderate proteins with healthy fats
- *Dinner:* Leaner protein choices to round out the day
- *Snack (optional):* Small bites for hunger or energy

Weekly Rotation by Weeks

Each week consists of rotating recipes to ensure variety and minimize cooking stress.

Week 1 Meal Plan

Day 1

- *Breakfast:* Scrambled eggs in duck fat (3 whole eggs) + 2 oz pork belly
- *Lunch:* Grilled chicken thighs (6 oz) with a dollop of butter
- *Dinner:* Salmon filet (6 oz) pan-seared in tallow
- *Snack:* Beef jerky (2 oz, no added sugar or carbs)

Day 2

- ***Breakfast:*** Boiled eggs (2 large) + 2 homemade sausage patties (3 oz patty each)
- ***Lunch:*** Sliced roast beef (5 oz) + bone broth (1 cup)
- ***Dinner:*** Grilled lamb chops (7 oz) with a drizzle of melted butter
- ***Snack:*** Pork rinds (1 handful)

Day 3

- ***Breakfast:*** Bacon (4 slices) + soft-boiled eggs (2 large)
- ***Lunch:*** Ribeye steak (8 oz, trimmed fat cooked separately)
- ***Dinner:*** Baked cod (6 oz) with ghee + chicken broth (1 cup)
- ***Snack:*** Smoked salmon (2 oz)

Day 4

- ***Breakfast:*** Omelette (3 eggs) with ground beef (2 oz)
- ***Lunch:*** Grilled chicken wings (6 pieces, skin-on) + bone broth (1 cup)
- ***Dinner:*** Pork tenderloin (6 oz) sautéed in butter
- ***Snack:*** Duck liver pâté (2 oz)

Day 5

- ***Breakfast:*** Hard-boiled eggs (3 large) with pork belly (3 oz)
- ***Lunch:*** Seared liver (4 oz) with scrambled eggs (2 large)

- ***Dinner:*** Bison burger (6 oz, no bun) + butter or ghee
- ***Snack:*** Sliced cheese (2 oz, optional for keto carnivore)

Day 6

- ***Breakfast:*** Grilled pork chops (5 oz) + 2 fried eggs
- ***Lunch:*** Roasted turkey (6 oz) with a side of bone marrow
- ***Dinner:*** Salmon steak (7 oz) drizzled with duck fat
- ***Snack:*** Beef tallow bites

Day 7

- ***Breakfast:*** Poached eggs (3 large) with a thin slice of smoked ham (3 oz)
- ***Lunch:*** Ribeye steak (8 oz) topped with a dollop of ghee
- ***Dinner:*** 80/20 ground beef patties (2 x 3 oz patties) grilled
- ***Snack:*** Pork crackling

Week 2–4 Plan Modifications

Repeat the recipes from Week 1, but switch up protein sources for variety. For example, replace chicken thighs with turkey legs, swap pork belly for lamb bacon, or try seafood like scallops or shrimp for dinners.

Sample Recipes

Light Baked Salmon

Ingredients:

- 6 oz salmon fillet
- 1 tbsp melted beef tallow
- Pinch of sea salt

Instructions:

1. Preheat the oven to 375°F.
2. Place salmon fillet on a baking sheet lined with parchment paper.
3. Brush melted beef tallow over the top of the salmon, then sprinkle with sea salt.
4. Bake for 10-12 minutes, or until desired level of doneness is reached.

Salmon Filet

Ingredients:

- 6 oz salmon fillet
- 1 tbsp melted beef tallow
- Pinch of sea salt

Instructions:

1. Heat a cast iron skillet over medium-high heat.
2. Brush the salmon fillet with melted beef tallow and sprinkle with sea salt.
3. Place the salmon in the heated skillet, skin side down.
4. Cook for about 4 minutes, then carefully flip the fillet over and cook for an additional 3-4 minutes, or until desired level of doneness is reached.
5. Serve hot and enjoy!

Carnivore Egg Muffins

Ingredients:

- 6 eggs
- 4 oz ground beef
- 1 tbsp butter (optional)

Instructions:

1. Preheat the oven to 375°F.
2. In a bowl, beat the eggs and set aside.
3. Cook ground beef in a pan until browned, then drain excess fat.
4. Add cooked ground beef to beaten eggs and mix well.
5. Grease muffin tin with butter (if desired) and pour egg mixture into each muffin cup.
6. Bake for 15 minutes or until eggs are fully cooked.

Crispy Pork Belly Strips

Ingredients:

- 5 oz pork belly
- Sea salt to taste

Instructions:

1. Preheat the oven to 375°F.
2. Place pork belly on a baking sheet lined with parchment paper.
3. Sprinkle sea salt over the top of the pork belly.
4. Bake for 20-25 minutes, or until pork belly is crispy and golden brown.

Tips for Staying Motivated

1. *Track Progress:* Keep a detailed log in a journal or use a fitness app to track weight, inches lost, or even energy levels over time. Seeing the improvements documented can keep you motivated and help you identify what's working best for you.
2. *Simplify Meal Prep:* Save time during busy weeks by doubling or tripling recipes when cooking. Store leftovers in portioned containers so you always have a healthy meal ready to go, avoiding the temptation of fast food or unhealthy snacks.
3. *Focus on Non-Scale Wins:* Progress isn't just about the number on the scale. Pay attention to other positive changes like clearer skin, reduced brain fog, improved digestion, or better sleep quality. These wins are just as important and show your efforts are paying off.
4. *Celebrate Small Wins:* Reward yourself for sticking to your goals, no matter how small the achievement. Treat yourself to a new kitchen gadget, a favorite ingredient, or even a relaxing activity to help maintain momentum and keep the journey enjoyable.

5. ***Hydration and Electrolytes:*** Staying hydrated is key for energy, focus, and overall health. Make sure to drink plenty of water throughout the day. Adding electrolytes, especially during increased physical activity, can help prevent fatigue, muscle cramps, and headaches.

This meal plan makes it easier to maintain a calorie deficit while enjoying nutrient-dense, satisfying meals. Stick with it for 30 days and adjust portions when needed for your goals.

30-Day High-Protein Carnivore Diet Muscle Building Meal Plan for Women

This meal plan is tailored for women aiming to build muscle and strength while following the carnivore diet. Rich in high-quality animal protein and healthy fats, it's structured for optimal muscle growth and recovery. The plan includes nutrient timing strategies to help maximize the benefits of workouts and detailed macronutrient guidance for each meal.

Nutrient Timing Strategies

To support muscle building, timing your meals around workouts is crucial.

- *Pre-Workout:* Consume a moderate-protein, moderate-fat meal 1–2 hours before training to fuel performance.
- *Post-Workout:* Within 30–60 minutes after your session, eat a high-protein meal with a small amount of fat to aid muscle recovery.

Macronutrient Ratios per Meal

- *Protein:* 1.2–1.5 grams per pound of lean body mass daily, distributed evenly across meals (around 30–40 grams per meal).
- *Fat:* 0.7–1.0 grams per pound of lean body mass to meet energy needs.

Example daily macro split for a 135-pound woman with an active goal to build muscle:

- Protein = 150 grams
- Fat = 105 grams

Meal Plan Overview

Each day includes Breakfast, Lunch, Dinner, and Snack (Post-Workout/Optional). Recipes rotate weekly to keep it varied and exciting, offering consistent progress in strength and recovery.

Week 1 Meal Plan

Day 1

- *Breakfast:* Ribeye steak (6 oz) + 2 fried eggs in butter (1 tbsp)

  Macros: 42g protein, 43g fat

- *Lunch (Pre-Workout):* Pork chops (6 oz) seared in lard (2 tbsp)

Macros: 39g protein, 48g fat

- **Snack (Post-Workout):** Bone broth (1 cup) + beef tenderloin (5 oz)

Macros: 35g protein, 12g fat

- **Dinner:** Grilled salmon (6 oz) topped with ghee (1 tbsp) + side of chicken broth

Macros: 38g protein, 20g fat

Day 2

- **Breakfast:** Ground bison patties (2 x 4 oz) + 2 scrambled eggs

Macros: 48g protein, 44g fat

- **Lunch (Pre-Workout):** Roasted lamb leg (7 oz) + 1 tbsp duck fat

Macros: 46g protein, 35g fat

- **Snack (Post-Workout):** Turkey breast (5 oz) with a slice of melted cheese (2 oz)

Macros: 40g protein, 13g fat

- **Dinner:** Pan-seared cod (6 oz) with shrimp (3 oz) in garlic butter (2 tbsp)

Macros: 45g protein, 19g fat

Day 3

- ***Breakfast:*** Scrambled eggs (3 large) in bacon grease + 4 slices of bacon

  Macros: 36g protein, 41g fat

- ***Lunch (Pre-Workout):*** Roasted bone marrow (2 large bones) + duck breast (5 oz)

  Macros: 32g protein, 42g fat

- ***Snack (Post-Workout):*** Sliced roast beef (5 oz) + 2 tbsp tallow

  Macros: 43g protein, 20g fat

- ***Dinner:*** Grilled elk steak (6 oz) + butter-sautéed chicken liver (2 oz)

  Macros: 40g protein, 22g fat

Day 4–7

Repeat meals from Days 1–3, modifying protein sources for variety (e.g., replace beef with venison or salmon with swordfish).

Week 2–4 Plan Adjustments

Rotate recipes from Week 1 with new options. Here are some alternate meals to introduce variety.

Breakfast Options

- ***Option 1:*** Lamb burger (6 oz) + fried eggs (2 large) cooked in duck fat

    Macros: 45g protein, 38g fat

- ***Option 2:*** Seared beef liver (4 oz) + bacon (3 slices)

    Macros: 42g protein, 40g fat

Lunch Options

- ***Option 1:*** Grilled swordfish (7 oz) + side of bone broth with butter (1 tbsp)

    Macros: 52g protein, 18g fat

- ***Option 2:*** Pork roast (6 oz) with a drizzle of rendered lard (1 tbsp)

    Macros: 40g protein, 36g fat

Dinner Options

- ***Option 1:*** Shrimp (8 oz) sautéed in garlic ghee (2 tbsp) + chicken broth on the side

    Macros: 42g protein, 16g fat

- ***Option 2:*** Roasted duck leg (6 oz) + crispy pork skin (2 oz)

    Macros: 48g protein, 23g fat

Snack (Post-Workout/Optional)

- *Option 1:* Boiled eggs (2 large) + pork belly (2 oz)

  Macros: 28g protein, 26g fat

- *Option 2:* Grilled chicken breast (6 oz) + a drizzle of melted ghee (1 tbsp)

  Macros: 39g protein, 10g fat

Sample Recipes

Roasted bone marrow

Ingredients:

- 2 lbs beef marrow bones
- Sea salt, to taste

Instructions:

1. Preheat oven to 450°F.
2. Place beef marrow bones on a baking sheet lined with foil.
3. Sprinkle sea salt over bones.
4. Roast for 15 minutes, or until the marrow is soft and bubbly.
5. Serve with a spoon and enjoy!

Grilled Swordfish

<u>Ingredients:</u>

- 1 lb swordfish steak
- Salt and pepper, to taste
- 2 tbsp ghee or butter, melted

<u>Instructions:</u>

1. Preheat grill to medium heat.
2. Season swordfish steak with salt and pepper on both sides.
3. Brush melted ghee or butter over the fish.
4. Grill for 5-6 minutes on each side, until fish flakes easily with a fork.
5. Serve hot and enjoy!

Seared Duck Breast

Ingredients:

- 6 oz duck breast
- Salt for seasoning

Instructions:

1. Score the skin of the duck breast with a sharp knife in a criss-cross pattern.
2. Season both sides of the duck breast generously with salt.
3. Heat a cast iron skillet over medium-high heat and place the duck breast, skin side down, on the pan.
4. Let it cook for 6-7 minutes until the skin is crispy and golden brown. Flip the duck breast and cook for an additional 3-4 minutes for medium-rare or longer for desired doneness.
5. Remove from heat and let it rest for 5 minutes before slicing and serving.

Bone Broth Protein Shot

Ingredients:

- 1 cup bone broth
- 1 tbsp butter

Instructions:

1. Heat bone broth in a saucepan over medium heat until simmering.
2. Remove from heat and stir in butter until fully melted.
3. Pour the mixture into a shot glass and enjoy as a protein-packed snack or post-workout drink.

Lamb Burgers

Ingredients:

- 8 oz ground lamb
- Sea salt

Instructions:

1. Preheat a grill or grill pan to medium-high heat.
2. Season ground lamb with sea salt and form into two equal-sized patties.
3. Cook patties for 5-6 minutes on each side, or until desired level of doneness is reached.
4. Serve on lettuce wraps or with your choice of toppings such as avocado, tomato, and onion.

Tips for Muscle Building Success

To achieve muscle building success, it's important to not only focus on your workouts but also pay attention to your nutrition and recovery. Here are some tips to help you reach your goals:

1. ***Prioritize Sleep:*** Recovery is essential for building strength and muscle, and it happens while you sleep. Aim for 7–8 hours of quality sleep each night to allow your body to repair and grow stronger. Create a consistent bedtime routine to ensure you're getting the rest you need.
2. ***Hydration is Key:*** Staying hydrated is crucial for optimal performance and recovery. Drink plenty of water throughout the day and replenish lost electrolytes, especially after intense workouts. Consider adding a hydration drink or electrolyte supplement if needed.
3. ***Track Progress:*** Keep an eye on your progress by measuring strength gains, muscle tone changes, and even energy levels on a weekly basis. Use a journal, app, or spreadsheet to document your lifts, reps, and any changes in body composition. Tracking helps you stay motivated and identify areas for improvement.
4. ***Stay Consistent:*** Follow the meal plan for at least 30 days to see real results. Adjust portions if needed to meet your energy requirements, but stick to the plan as

closely as possible. Consistency with both nutrition and training is key to achieving your goals.
5. ***Lift Heavy:*** Focus on progressive overload in your strength training routine to continually challenge your muscles. Gradually increase the weight, reps, or intensity to build strength and muscle over time. Remember to maintain proper form to prevent injuries and maximize gains.

Follow this high-protein, muscle-building carnivore diet for a full month, and watch your strength and physique transform while enjoying nutrient-dense meals that fuel performance and recovery.

14-Day Carnivore Diet Meal Plan for Energy and Focus

The Carnivore Diet can amplify mental clarity and energy when paired with the right nutrient-dense foods. For busy professionals, it's essential to prioritize meals rich in brain-boosting nutrients like omega-3 fatty acids, choline, and B vitamins, while keeping them quick and easy to prepare. Below is a 14-day meal plan designed for sustained energy and improved focus, tailored to fit into a hectic schedule.

Key Nutrients for Energy and Focus

To stay energized and focused throughout the day, it's important to prioritize foods rich in the following nutrients:

1. *Omega-3 Fatty Acids:* Found in fatty fish like salmon, sardines, and mackerel, omega-3s support brain function and reduce mental fatigue.
2. *Choline:* Eggs and organ meats, particularly the liver, are excellent sources of choline, critical for memory and cognitive performance.

3. ***B Vitamins:*** Beef, chicken, and liver are rich in B vitamins, which help convert food into energy and support proper brain activity.
4. ***Iron:*** Essential for oxygen transport to the brain, iron from red meat promotes sustained focus and prevents fatigue.
5. ***Healthy Fats:*** Grass-fed butter, tallow, and ghee provide dense energy sources for a low-carb, brain-friendly fuel supply.

By incorporating these key nutrients into your meals, you'll notice a significant improvement in energy and focus.

Meal Guidelines for Busy Professionals

Efficient meal planning is essential for busy professionals striving to maintain steady energy, maximize productivity, and simplify their daily routines.

- ***Simple and Quick:*** These meals are designed to save you time, requiring fewer than 30 minutes to prepare. They incorporate batch cooking methods and straightforward recipes, making them perfect for busy schedules while still delivering delicious and nutritious results.
- ***Portion Control:*** Proper portioning is key to meeting your dietary needs. These meals are easy to adjust based on your daily energy requirements, which for most professionals with moderate physical activity

typically range between ~1,800–2,200 calories. This helps ensure you're fueling your body without overeating or feeling sluggish.
- *Meal Timing:* Strategically plan two to three balanced meals per day to keep your energy levels steady. This approach avoids the post-lunch energy crashes that can impact productivity, keeping you focused and energized throughout the day.

By following these simple meal guidelines, you can fuel your body, support a balanced lifestyle, and stay energized to tackle the demands of your day effectively.

14-Day Meal Plan

Week 1
Day 1

- *Breakfast:* 3 pasture-raised eggs scrambled in 1 tbsp grass-fed butter, 2 oz smoked salmon.
- *Lunch:* 7 oz seared salmon with 1 tbsp tallow, a side of bone broth (1 cup).
- *Dinner:* 8 oz grass-fed ribeye steak cooked in its own fat.

Day 2

- *Breakfast:* 2 hard-boiled eggs, 1 oz pork rinds for crunch.

- *Lunch:* 6 oz grilled chicken thighs with 1 tbsp ghee.
- *Dinner:* 7 oz pan-fried mackerel with a drizzle of butter.

Day 3

- *Breakfast:* 3 sunny-side-up eggs cooked in tallow, 2 oz thinly sliced liver for choline boost.
- *Lunch:* 7 oz turkey breast with rendered fat drizzle and a cup of bone broth.
- *Dinner:* 8 oz lamb chops with 1 tsp sea salt.

Day 4

- *Breakfast:* 3 egg omelette with diced beef liver (1 oz) and 1 tbsp butter.
- *Lunch:* 6 oz beef patties with melted cheddar cheese (optional).
- *Dinner:* 7 oz broiled sardines with 1 tbsp olive oil drizzle.

Day 5

- *Breakfast:* 2 poached eggs with 3 oz smoked salmon and 1 tbsp avocado oil (optional for omega-3 boost).
- *Lunch:* 6 oz chicken breast with 1 tsp bacon grease.
- *Dinner:* 8 oz seared cod with 1 tbsp melted ghee.

Day 6

- ***Breakfast:*** 3 scrambled eggs with a pinch of salt and 2 oz grilled liver.
- ***Lunch:*** 7 oz pork chops cooked in tallow with a side of bone broth.
- ***Dinner:*** 8 oz grass-fed ground beef stir-fried in tallow.

Day 7

- ***Breakfast:*** Simple breakfast of 3 fried eggs in ghee.
- ***Lunch:*** 6 oz grilled salmon with lemon butter sauce.
- ***Dinner:*** 7 oz roasted duck breast with 1 tbsp rendered fat.

Week 2

Day 8

- ***Breakfast:*** 2 boiled eggs with 1 oz prosciutto slices.
- ***Lunch:*** 7 oz beef patties mixed with 2 oz diced liver.
- ***Dinner:*** 8 oz snapper fillets cooked in tallow, seasoned with salt.

Day 9

- ***Breakfast:*** Omelette with 3 eggs, 2 oz canned sardines, and a drizzle of butter.
- ***Lunch:*** 7 oz seared chicken thighs and 1 cup of bone broth.
- ***Dinner:*** 9 oz lamb chops cooked in rendered fat.

Day 10

- *Breakfast:* 3 scrambled eggs with 1 oz melted feta cheese (optional).
- *Lunch:* 6 oz turkey breast with 1 tbsp bacon grease.
- *Dinner:* 8 oz baked salmon drizzled with ghee.

Day 11

- *Breakfast:* 3 fried eggs with a side of ground pork (4 oz).
- *Lunch:* 7 oz grilled bison steak with bone broth (1 cup).
- *Dinner:* 8 oz broiled cod served with 1 tbsp grass-fed butter.

Day 12

- *Breakfast:* 2 boiled eggs, 3 oz liver sausage slices.
- *Lunch:* 7 oz beef patties topped with melted cheddar (optional).
- *Dinner:* 8 oz roasted trout cooked with tallow.

Day 13

- *Breakfast:* Omelette with 3 eggs and 2 oz diced chicken breast.
- *Lunch:* 6 oz seared duck breast with 1 tbsp duck fat.
- *Dinner:* 8 oz grass-fed ribeye steak with a side of bone broth.

Day 14

- *Breakfast:* 3 scrambled eggs cooked in tallow.
- *Lunch:* 7 oz grilled lamb steak with melted butter drizzle.
- *Dinner:* 9 oz pan-fried salmon cooked in bacon grease.

Quick Recipes for Busy Days

5-Minute Sardine Snack

Ingredients:

- 1 can of sardines (packed in water or olive oil)
- 1 tsp lemon juice (optional)

Instructions:

1. Drain the water or oil from the sardines.
2. Place sardines on a plate and drizzle with lemon juice, if desired.
3. Enjoy as a quick protein-packed snack!

Simple Ribeye

Ingredients:

- 8 oz ribeye steak
- 1 tsp salt

Instructions:

1. Preheat a cast iron skillet on high heat.
2. Sprinkle salt over both sides of the steak.
3. Place the steak in the hot skillet and cook for 4 minutes on each side (for medium-rare).
4. Let it rest for a few minutes before serving.

Hard-Boiled Egg Prep

Ingredients:

- 6–12 pasture-raised eggs

Instructions:

1. Fill a pot with enough water to cover the eggs.
2. Bring the water to a boil, then reduce heat to low and gently place the eggs in the pot.
3. Cook for 8 minutes for soft-boiled or 12 minutes for hard-boiled.
4. Drain hot water and immediately place eggs in cold water to stop cooking process.
5. Peel and store in an airtight container in the fridge for quick and easy snacks throughout the week.

Liver Boost Stir-Fry

Ingredients:

- 6 oz ground beef
- 2 oz diced liver
- 1 tbsp ghee

Instructions:

1. Heat ghee in a pan over medium heat.
2. Add ground beef and liver, stirring occasionally until fully cooked.
3. Serve with your choice of vegetables for a quick and nutrient-dense stir-fry meal.

Banana Almond Smoothie

Ingredients:

- 1 ripe banana
- 1 cup unsweetened almond milk
- 2 tbsp almond butter
- 1 tsp honey (optional)

Instructions:

1. Combine all ingredients in a blender.
2. Blend until smooth and creamy.
3. Serve immediately for a nutritious and delicious snack or breakfast option.

Final Tips for Energy and Focus

- ***Batch Cook:*** Prepare meals like boiled eggs, beef patties, and bone broth in advance to save time during the workweek.
- ***Stay Hydrated:*** Drink plenty of water and include bone broth for added minerals and electrolytes.
- ***Mindful Portions:*** Adjust meal sizes and spacing to align with your hunger and activity levels throughout the day.

This plan not only supports sustained energy and mental clarity but also fits seamlessly into a busy lifestyle. With these quick, nutrient-dense meals, you'll stay sharp, productive, and energized all day long!

21-Day Carnivore Diet Meal Plan for Anti-Aging and Skin Health

The Carnivore Diet can be a powerful tool for promoting anti-aging and skin health. By focusing on foods rich in collagen, omega-3 fatty acids, and other skin-nourishing nutrients, you can support elasticity, hydration, and a youthful glow. This 21-day meal plan will guide you toward healthy, glowing skin while emphasizing strategies to reduce sugar-induced skin aging.

Key Nutrients for Anti-Aging and Glowing Skin

1. *Collagen:* Found in bone broth, chicken skin, and connective tissues, collagen helps maintain skin elasticity and firmness.
2. *Omega-3 Fatty Acids:* Fatty fish like salmon, mackerel, and sardines provide omega-3s that reduce inflammation and promote skin hydration.
3. *Vitamin A:* The liver is rich in vitamin A, essential for cell turnover and reducing signs of aging, like fine lines and wrinkles.

4. ***Zinc:*** Found in red meat and shellfish, zinc helps repair skin damage and combat acne.
5. ***Healthy Fats:*** Fats from grass-fed butter, tallow, and ghee support a glowing complexion and reduce inflammation.
6. ***Low-Carb Focus:*** By reducing sugar and carbs, the Carnivore Diet minimizes glycation, a process that accelerates skin aging by breaking down collagen and elastin.

Tips for Reducing Sugar-Induced Skin Aging

- ***Stick to Zero-Sugar Foods:*** Eliminate high-sugar snacks and focus solely on animal products to avoid spikes in blood sugar that damage your skin.
- ***Hydrate with Bone Broth:*** Bone broth not only hydrates but also delivers collagen and amino acids to support skin repair.
- ***Avoid Processed Meats:*** Stick to whole, unprocessed cuts of meat to ensure your meals are nutrient-dense and free from inflammatory additives.
- ***Include Omega-3s Daily:*** Fatty fish should be a regular part of your meal plan to keep skin supple and moist.

21-Day Anti-Aging Meal Plan

Week 1

Day 1

- *Breakfast:* 3 boiled eggs with 2 oz crispy chicken skin for collagen.
- *Lunch:* 7 oz grilled salmon with 1 tbsp butter.
- *Dinner:* 8 oz bone-in ribeye steak cooked in tallow, a small side of bone broth (1 cup).

Day 2

- *Breakfast:* Omelette with 3 eggs and 1 oz diced liver for vitamin A boost.
- *Lunch:* 6 oz mackerel with a drizzle of ghee.
- *Dinner:* 7 oz lamb chops cooked with 1 tbsp rendered fat.

Day 3

- *Breakfast:* Scrambled eggs (2 whole, 1 extra yolk) cooked in butter.
- *Lunch:* 7 oz baked cod with collagen-rich skin left on.
- *Dinner:* 8 oz slow-cooked beef shank with a side of bone broth.

Day 4

- *Breakfast:* 2 poached eggs with 3 oz smoked salmon.
- *Lunch:* 6 oz pork belly with crispy skin.

- **Dinner:** 7 oz roasted duck breast with 1 tbsp rendered duck fat.

Day 5

- **Breakfast:** 3 fried eggs in bacon grease, 2 oz bacon (uncured).
- **Lunch:** 7 oz grilled turkey leg.
- **Dinner:** 9 oz braised oxtail for collagen-rich goodness.

Day 6

- **Breakfast:** Hard-boiled eggs (x3) with 1 oz liver sausage.
- **Lunch:** 6 oz grilled sardines with a drizzle of olive oil (optional omega-3 boost).
- **Dinner:** 8 oz grass-fed beef patties with bone broth.

Day 7

- **Breakfast:** 3 scrambled eggs with diced salmon roe for omega-3s.
- **Lunch:** 6 oz turkey breast cooked in butter with crispy skin.
- **Dinner:** 7 oz braised beef short ribs with collagen-rich broth.

Week 2

Day 8

- **Breakfast:** 2 boiled eggs with 1 oz prosciutto.

- *Lunch:* 6 oz baked trout, seasoned with sea salt.
- *Dinner:* 8 oz grilled lamb steak with melted tallow.

Day 9

- *Breakfast:* 3 fried eggs with 1 oz diced liver.
- *Lunch:* 7 oz bone-in chicken thighs, cooked crispy.
- *Dinner:* 8 oz pan-seared mackerel with ghee drizzle.

Day 10

- *Breakfast:* Omelette with 2 whole eggs and 2 oz bone marrow chunks.
- *Lunch:* 6 oz roast turkey neck for collagen boost.
- *Dinner:* 8 oz broiled salmon with 1 tbsp melted butter.

Day 11

- *Breakfast:* 3 sunny-side-up eggs with 1 oz smoked salmon.
- *Lunch:* 6 oz sardines with olive oil drizzle (optional).
- *Dinner:* 8 oz grilled bison steak with bone broth side.

Day 12

- *Breakfast:* 2 egg omelette with 1 oz crispy chicken skin.
- *Lunch:* 7 oz seared duck breast with rendered fat.
- *Dinner:* 9 oz braised pork shoulder with gelatin-rich broth.

Day 13

- *Breakfast:* 3 boiled eggs with 2 oz beef liver.
- *Lunch:* 7 oz baked cod with plenty of skin.
- *Dinner:* 8 oz beef stew featuring shanks and marrow bones.

Day 14

- *Breakfast:* 2 poached eggs with 3 oz sardines.
- *Lunch:* 6 oz turkey breast with tallow for fat boost.
- *Dinner:* 7 oz grilled salmon and 1 cup of collagen-heavy bone broth.

Week 3

Day 15

- *Breakfast:* Scrambled eggs (2 whole, 1 yolk) with butter.
- *Lunch:* 6 oz lamb shank in its own broth.
- *Dinner:* 8 oz grass-fed ribeye steak topped with tallow.

Day 16

- *Breakfast:* 2 fried eggs with 2 oz liver pâté.
- *Lunch:* 6 oz mackerel cooked in ghee.
- *Dinner:* 8 oz braised pork belly.

Day 17

- *Breakfast:* 3 hard-boiled eggs with 1 tbsp mayo (optional).
- *Lunch:* 7 oz sardines for omega-3 boost.

- ***Dinner:*** 9 oz roasted chicken drumsticks with crispy skin.

Day 18

- ***Breakfast:*** Omelette with 3 eggs and 2 oz smoked salmon.
- ***Lunch:*** 6 oz grilled lamb chops with tallow drippings.
- ***Dinner:*** 8 oz baked trout, skin on.

Day 19

- ***Breakfast:*** Scrambled eggs (2 whole, 1 yolk) cooked in bacon grease.
- ***Lunch:*** 7 oz roasted turkey wings for collagen content.
- ***Dinner:*** 8 oz slow-cooked beef cheeks with a side of bone broth.

Day 20

- ***Breakfast:*** 3 eggs (fried in tallow) with 2 oz salmon roe.
- ***Lunch:*** 8 oz baked salmon with butter drizzle.
- ***Dinner:*** 9 oz roasted lamb with rendered fat.

Day 21

- ***Breakfast:*** 2 boiled eggs with sardines in olive oil (optional).
- ***Lunch:*** 6 oz ground bison patties topped with cheddar (optional).
- ***Dinner:*** 8 oz roasted duck leg with broth.

Recipes for Skin Health

Simple Bone Broth

Ingredients:

- 2 lbs beef or chicken bones
- Water to cover
- 1 tbsp apple cider vinegar

Instructions:

1. Place bones in a large pot and cover with water.
2. Add apple cider vinegar and let sit for 20-30 minutes.
3. Bring to a boil, then reduce heat and simmer for at least 12 hours (up to 24 hours) on low heat.
4. Skim off any impurities that rise to the surface.
5. Let broth cool, then strain through a fine mesh strainer or cheesecloth.
6. Store in an airtight container in the fridge for up to one week or freeze for longer storage.

Crispy Chicken Skin Chips

Ingredients:

- Chicken skin from 1 whole chicken
- Sea salt

Instructions:

1. Preheat oven to 375°F (190°C).
2. Place chicken skin on a parchment-lined baking sheet.
3. Sprinkle with sea salt.
4. Bake for 15-20 minutes, or until the skin is crispy and golden brown.
5. Let cool and enjoy as a snack or use as a topping for salads or soups.

Seared Salmon with Butter

Ingredients:

- 6 oz salmon filet
- 1 tbsp grass-fed butter

Instructions:

1. Heat a skillet over medium-high heat.
2. Add butter and let it melt.
3. Place salmon filet skin-side down in the skillet.
4. Cook for 4-5 minutes, then flip and cook for an additional 2-3 minutes (or until desired doneness).
5. Serve with your choice of vegetables or enjoy on its own.

Final Tips for Glowing Skin

To keep your skin healthy and glowing, here are a few additional tips to keep in mind:

- *Hydrate Regularly:* Drink plenty of water throughout the day to keep your skin hydrated and support overall health. Consider adding hydrating foods like fruits and vegetables or incorporating broth-based soups to further combat dehydration. Proper hydration helps maintain skin elasticity and reduce dryness.
- *Get Quality Sleep:* Aim for 7-9 hours of quality sleep each night to allow your body to repair itself. During sleep, collagen production increases, which is essential for maintaining firm, youthful skin. Adequate rest also reduces inflammation, dark circles, and puffiness, ensuring a healthy glow.
- *Stay Consistent:* Stick to this plan daily to see lasting improvements in your skin's health and appearance. Remember, skincare is a long-term commitment, and consistency is key to achieving and maintaining vibrant, healthy skin.

This 21-day plan targets anti-aging and skin health with nutrient-dense, easy-to-make meals. Stick with it, and enjoy a healthier, more youthful glow!

Inspiring Success Stories from Women on the Carnivore Diet

Judy

Judy Cho's journey with the carnivore diet transformed her life and her family's health. After years of struggling with major depression and an eating disorder, she found healing through a meat-based diet.

Judy shares, "Carnivore is a lifeline that standard care never gave as an option." Her parents, once plagued by diabetes and other health issues, also experienced remarkable improvements. Judy's story highlights the potential of the carnivore diet to offer hope and healing, emphasizing that while it may not be for everyone, it can be a powerful tool for those seeking change.

Alisha Khan

Alisha Khan, a wellness coach from Toronto, transformed her life with a low-carb, high-fat carnivore diet and intermittent fasting. Struggling with chronic pain and weight issues, she found relief and lost 35 pounds.

Alisha shares, "I adore this way of eating because it allows me to eat foods that taste incredible, while helping me lose weight, keeping me satiated, and reducing pain symptoms." Her journey emphasizes the importance of self-love and community support. Alisha's story inspires others to embrace change, highlighting that health and self-worth are achievable with the right mindset and lifestyle.

Barb Shaw

Barb Shaw, 53, embraced the carnivore diet after years of experimenting with various eating styles. Raised on a low-fat diet, she and her husband tried veganism and keto before discovering carnivore. Barb shares, "My GI tract is doing so well, and my rash cleared up in a matter of weeks."

The diet improved her energy, sleep, and muscle tone, while her husband reduced his blood pressure medication. Despite initial skepticism, Barb found satisfaction in the simplicity and effectiveness of the carnivore lifestyle, highlighting its potential to enhance health and well-being without the need for plant-based foods.

Conclusion

Congratulations on making it to the end of this Carnivore Meal Plan and Grocery Guide for Women! Taking the time to educate yourself about a new way of nourishing your body is no small feat. You've just empowered yourself with practical tools—from meal plans to grocery shopping tips and kitchen essentials—to successfully embrace the carnivore lifestyle. Take a moment to celebrate because you've set yourself up for success in a way that few people do.

Making the decision to simplify your diet is as courageous as it is exciting. Shifting to a carnivore diet means cutting through the noise of endless food choices and reconnecting with fundamentals. It's not just a diet but a lifestyle—a way to avoid inflammatory foods and focus on nutrient-dense meals that fuel your body and mind. Whether your goal is weight loss, hormone balance, glowing skin, or improved strength, you now have a clear roadmap to get you there.

That said, the carnivore diet isn't without its challenges. It's normal to encounter moments of doubt, especially when faced with the restrictive nature of the diet or social situations where animal-based eating may feel isolating. But remember this—isn't it worth exploring something that could change the way you feel, think, and live? If challenges arise, lean into solutions. Plan ahead, stay prepared, and always keep your "why" front and center. Whether you're doing this for more energy, better clarity, or simply to take control of your health, that motivation will keep you moving forward.

Think of this guide as your companion for both the exciting days when the results start coming in and the tough days when motivation feels distant. Use the meal plans as a tool to avoid decision fatigue, the grocery guide to streamline shopping, and the tips scattered throughout to troubleshoot any obstacles. Each meal you prepare, every time you check the inventory on your freezer's cuts of meat, and each steak you sear to perfection is a step closer to your goals.

It's also worth remembering that you're not alone in this. Women around the world have turned to the carnivore diet to reclaim their health with great success. They, too, started as beginners, using meal plans, refining their approach, and learning what works through experience. Take comfort in their victories, knowing that your success is just as reachable.

Now is the time to put what you've learned into action. Start with small, consistent steps. Build your first week of meals, prep your pantry, and shop smarter. If results don't come overnight, be patient with yourself. This is a long-term lifestyle—one where sustainable progress beats perfection every time.

Most importantly, trust that you're making choices that serve you. The path you've begun is not about avoiding food but about fully nourishing your body in ways that make you thrive. Stay curious, stay determined, and enjoy the process of transformation. You're fueling more than your appetite—you're building a better you.

FAQs

What is the carnivore diet, and how does it work?

The carnivore diet focuses exclusively on animal-based foods like meat, fish, eggs, and animal fats, while excluding all plant-based foods. By eliminating carbohydrates, your body shifts to using fat as its primary energy source, entering a state called ketosis. This can lead to stable energy levels, reduced cravings, and other potential health benefits.

What are the main benefits of the carnivore diet for women?

Women may experience hormonal balance, improved weight management, enhanced energy levels, better mental clarity, and healthier skin and joints. By eliminating inflammatory foods, the diet can also help regulate insulin levels and reduce symptoms of PCOS or irregular cycles. It's essential to focus on nutrient-dense foods for the best results.

How do I plan meals without feeling bored or deprived?

To avoid monotony, rotate different protein sources such as beef, chicken, lamb, pork, seafood, and organ meats. Use a variety of cooking methods like grilling, slow cooking, or pan-searing to keep meals exciting. Incorporating high-quality fats like tallow, ghee, and butter can add flavor while boosting your energy levels.

Is it expensive to follow the carnivore diet?

It doesn't have to be. You can save money by buying in bulk, focusing on budget-friendly cuts like ground beef or pork shoulder, and seeking deals at farmers' markets or local butchers. Including organ meats, which are nutrient-dense and affordable, is another cost-effective strategy. Frozen options and bulk online orders are also helpful for controlling costs.

How do I address potential nutrient deficiencies?

While the diet excludes plant foods, focusing on a variety of animal-based options can cover most nutritional needs. Include organ meats like liver for vitamins A and B12, fatty fish for omega-3s, and bone broth for collagen and minerals. Adequate hydration and electrolyte supplementation can also prevent imbalances, especially during the adaptation phase.

What challenges might I face on the carnivore diet?

Initial challenges may include fatigue, cravings, and digestive changes as your body adjusts to fewer carbs. Social situations and meal variety can also feel restrictive. Planning ahead, meal prepping, and staying consistent can help. If necessary, ease into the diet gradually instead of making an abrupt shift.

Can I adapt this diet to fit my health goals (e.g., weight loss or muscle building)?

Absolutely! The guide includes tailored meal plans for different goals such as weight loss, muscle building, energy, and skincare. Adjust portion sizes, protein-to-fat ratios, and meal timing to support goals like fat loss, strength gains, or improved focus. Always prioritize consistency and nutrient-dense foods for the best results.

References and Helpful Links

Watson, S. (2024, August 26). Carnivore diet: meal plan, food list, and what you should know. WebMD. https://www.webmd.com/diet/carnivore-diet

Sweenie, J. (2024, November 20). Top 5 benefits of a carnivore diet for Women - MyPrimalCoach. myPrimalCoach. https://www.myprimalcoach.com/blog/carnivore-diet-for-women/

Pursuit, I., & Pursuit, I. (2023, August 18). Carnivore diet food list: What should you grab at the grocery store? Carnivore Snax. https://carnivoresnax.com/blogs/articles/carnivore-diet-food-list?srsltid=AfmBOopMJFOZtYQRwufFCNxJ5gp9fLytCiiICzn4e_vmhOC8aAvFeayN

Judy, N. W. (2024, June 28). How the Carnivore Diet Changed Our Lives | Nutrition with Judy. Nutrition With Judy. https://www.nutritionwithjudy.com/how-carnivore-diet-healed-my-family

Clinic, C. (2024a, June 14). A beginner's guide to healthy meal prep. Cleveland Clinic. https://health.clevelandclinic.org/a-beginners-guide-to-healthy-meal-prep

Ld, L. S. M. R. (2024b, May 29). All you need to know about the carnivore (All-Meat) diet. Healthline. https://www.healthline.com/nutrition/carnivore-diet

The Carnivore Diet for Women: Female-Specific Effects and Benefits - Dr. Robert Kiltz. (2023, December 20). Dr. Robert Kiltz. https://www.doctorkiltz.com/carnivore-diet-for-women/

www.ingramcontent.com/pod-product-compliance
Lightning Source LLC
LaVergne TN
LVHW012029060526
838201LV00061B/4531